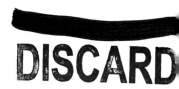

Everything
You Need to
Know About

Cystic
Fibrosis

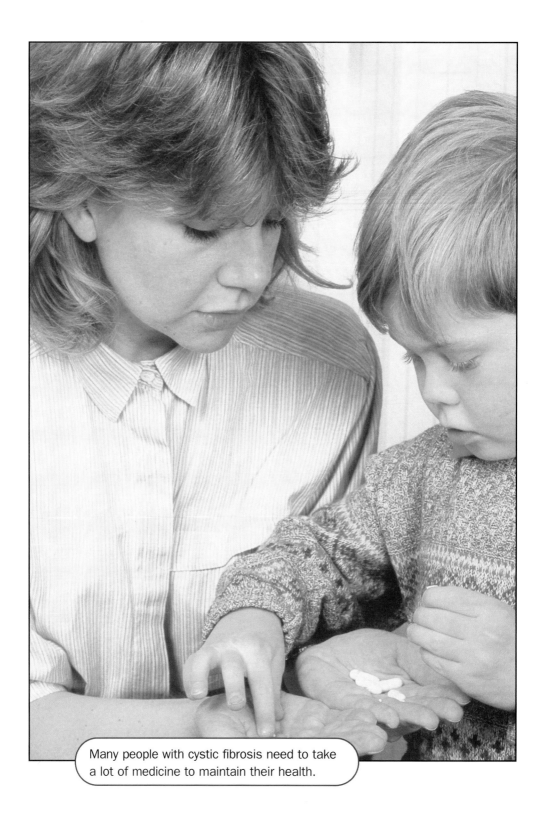
Many people with cystic fibrosis need to take a lot of medicine to maintain their health.

Everything You Need to Know About

Cystic Fibrosis

Justin Lee

The Rosen Publishing Group, Inc.
New York

To the Brown family. They have taught me so much about this disease, and they are a source of hope and inspiration.

Published in 2001 by The Rosen Publishing Group, Inc.
29 East 21st Street, New York, NY 10010

First Edition

Library of Congress Cataloging-in-Publication Data

Lee, Justin
    Everything you need to know about cystic fibrosis / Justin Lee. — 1st ed.
        p. cm. — (The need to know library)
Includes bibliographical references (p.   ) and index.
    ISBN 0-8239-3321-0 (library binding)
    1. Cystic fibrosis—Juvenile literature. [1. Cystic fibrosis. 2. Diseases.] I. Title. II. Series.
    RC858.C95 L44 2000
    616.3'7—dc21

                                                    00-010115

Manufactured in the United States of America

Contents

Introduction

Meggie wasn't thinking about social studies or the test that she had to take. She was thinking about her friend Alex who was in the hospital. Alex has cystic fibrosis, and she has to do many things to take care of herself that most other people don't have to do. One of those things is going to the hospital sometimes when she gets a cold. She has to take special medicine and do special exercises. She also has to eat a lot more than most people.

Meggie was looking down at her test and reading over the questions when she heard the door open. Alex walked in and sat down at her desk. Meggie looked over at her and Alex smiled. Mr. Korcy came over and talked to Alex for a moment, asking her if she was ready for the test *or if she wanted another couple of days because she had been sick. Alex said that she was ready. That was the way Alex was, she never needed to catch up. She was smart and always got good grades. Whenever she was in the hospital, she came back to school way ahead of everyone else. Meggie didn't understand it, but Alex said that it was because it was boring in the hospital.*

It isn't uncommon for people with cystic fibrosis to have to stay in the hospital to receive the special care that they need. Cystic fibrosis, or CF, is a very serious disease. It causes the lungs to get clogged up, making breathing difficult. People who have it are also more likely to get respiratory infections, meaning that hospital stays may last even longer.

About 30,000 Americans have CF. Another 3,000 people in Canada suffer from this disease. It is more common in Caucasians and African Americans than in Asians and Native Americans. CF is a genetic disease, meaning that it is passed on to you from your parents. This book will tell you why some people have CF and how they got it. It will also tell you some of the ways that you can deal with this disease. With new treatments, people with CF are living longer, healthier lives. Many people with the disease are living into their fifties. Only thirty years ago, that was unheard of—most people with CF died before the age of eighteen.

This book will go over the things you can do to help yourself if you have CF. It will also let you know what to expect if a friend or sibling has this disease. It is important to remember that people with CF are just like the rest of us. They love to play sports, socialize, have boyfriends and girlfriends, and do all the things that you and I like to do. You can't catch CF, so don't worry about that. If you have cystic fibrosis, or know someone who does, or just want to know more about this disease, read on.

Chapter One | What Is Cystic Fibrosis and How Does It Work?

Cystic fibrosis is a fatal disease. Like the rest of us, everyone who has cystic fibrosis will eventually die. However, those with CF have to work a lot harder to stay healthy.

A Salty Problem

We crave salty foods because our bodies need salt. The chemical formula for salt is NaCl. Salt is made up of sodium and chloride. "Na" is the symbol for sodium and "Cl" is the symbol for chloride. People with CF have a problem dealing with chloride.

Chloride is found in many cells in the body. The cells control how much chloride they have in them by letting some in and pushing excess chloride out. The cells of people without CF produce a protein called CFTR. This protein allows chloride ions to pass in and out of cells.

If this is confusing, try to visualize a tunnel under a river. Without the tunnel, people can't drive from one side of the river to the other. CFTR is a tunnel through the walls of the body's cells. If it is missing, chloride ions can't pass through the cell walls.

People with cystic fibrosis don't produce CFTR. When chloride can't pass through the cell walls, the mucus of the body becomes very thick and sticky. In people with CF, the mucus is what causes the problems in the lungs and the intestines. People with CF can't reabsorb the salt that they sweat out, and they become dehydrated faster than most people do.

Problems in the Lungs

Our lungs allow us to breathe. We can't survive more than a couple of minutes without breathing. With every breath we take, our lungs bring oxygen into our bodies and push out harmful carbon dioxide. Air rushes into our respiratory systems through our mouths or our noses. It then heads down our windpipes. These muscular tubes branch off into smaller and smaller tubes. These small tubes finally end in very tiny little sacs called alveoli. There are more than 300 million alveoli in our lungs. It is in these tiny sacs that oxygen is absorbed into our blood and carbon dioxide is pushed out.

The respiratory system is mostly made up of epithelial, or skin, cells. Spread out among these skin cells are

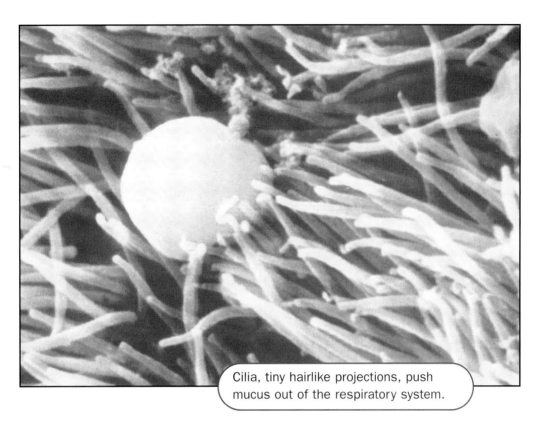

Cilia, tiny hairlike projections, push mucus out of the respiratory system.

mucous cells, which secrete a thin substance called mucus. Mucus protects the respiratory system by keeping it lubricated. It also traps any germs that may make their way down into the lungs. Cilia—tiny hair-like projections in the respiratory system—push the mucus up and out. From there it is sneezed or coughed out of the body. Sometimes the mucus is swallowed. Once it gets to the stomach, strong digestive acids kill any germs it might be carrying. Eventually the mucus is passed through the intestines and is excreted.

The mucus of people with cystic fibrosis has an unusually high amount of salt in it. Salty mucus is thicker and stickier than normal mucus, making it harder for the respiratory system to push it up and out. Thick mucus blocks the airways, making it harder to breathe. When airways are blocked, people may cough a lot because their bodies are trying to clear the passageways. If the body can't get the airways clear, the alveoli can start to get inflamed or swollen, making it even harder to breathe. If this condition worsens, eventually the lungs can collapse.

Another problem with salty mucus is that it makes it harder for the body's white blood cells to find and kill the germs that make their way down into the respiratory system. People with CF have a problem with respiratory infections because their bodies have a harder time killing these germs. When a person with CF gets a respiratory infection, the body tries to fight it by producing more mucus, which actually makes the problem worse.

All of these problems make it hard for people with cystic fibrosis to keep their lungs healthy. If these problems aren't solved, they will eventually kill the CF sufferer. That is why people with CF need to take extra special care of their lungs.

Problems with the Digestive System

Although respiratory problems are the greatest danger to a person with CF, another serious problem is the potential ineffectiveness of the digestive system. The digestive system is basically a long tube that starts at

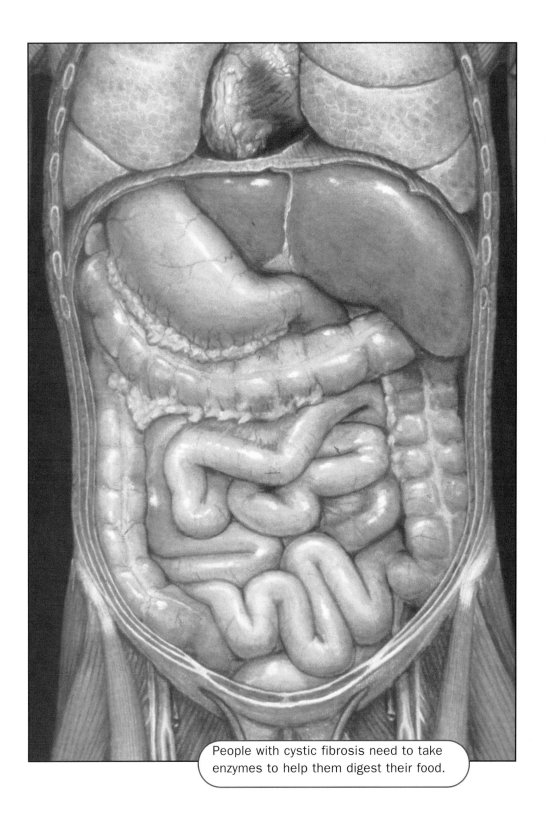

People with cystic fibrosis need to take enzymes to help them digest their food.

the mouth and ends where waste products leave the body. At different points along that tube, food is chewed up, broken down, torn apart, and absorbed into the bloodstream. The blood then carries the important nutrients to all parts of the body. When food leaves the stomach, it enters the intestine. There it is broken down even further by enzymes and bile. The enzymes come from an organ called the pancreas. The bile comes from the liver. The pancreas produces a group of enzymes that break down food (fat, proteins, and starches) for the body to use. The average person's pancreas weighs about three ounces. That may seem small, but the pancreas produces about thirty-two ounces of enzymes a day—more than ten times its own weight.

With CF sufferers, mucus clogs the small tubes that lead out of the pancreas. The enzymes that would normally break down the food never reach it. Eventually the pancreas can become scarred and may stop producing enzymes as well as it used to. When the food isn't broken down properly, the body can't absorb the nutrients it needs. Instead of nourishing the body, the food passes out of the body as unused waste. People with CF need to take enzymes to help digest their food because their natural enzymes can't reach the food.

Sometimes mucus also blocks the ducts leading out of the liver. When this happens, bile can't get to the intestine to break down the fats, and the liver can scar and stop functioning properly. This is called cirrhosis.

Chapter Two

How Do You Get Cystic Fibrosis?

Cystic fibrosis is a genetic disease, meaning that it is passed from parents to their children through genes.

It's in the Genes

Genes are the blueprints for the cells in our bodies. Our bodies have millions of different genes, which are stored on our chromosomes. Each person has twenty-three pairs of chromosomes—one set of twenty-three from each parent. These chromosomes pair up with each other, meaning that, for example, the hair gene from your father pairs up with the hair gene from your mother.

Our chromosomes contain all the information our bodies need to make cells and do all the things that bodies need to do. Cystic fibrosis is a problem with

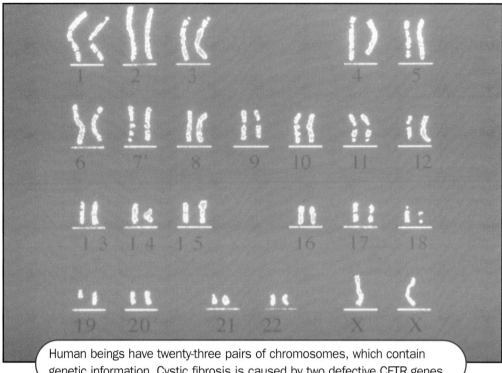

Human beings have twenty-three pairs of chromosomes, which contain genetic information. Cystic fibrosis is caused by two defective CFTR genes.

one specific gene. In 1985, scientists discovered that the CF gene is located on chromosome 7. Even though they knew what chromosome it was on, they didn't find which specific gene it was until 1989. That is because there are so many genes on each chromosome.

When scientists discovered the gene that is responsible for CF, what they really discovered is a normal gene that is defective in some people. The gene is called the CFTR gene. CFTR stands for cystic fibrosis transmembrane conductance regulator. This gene tells the body how to make a certain protein (also called CFTR), which is made in the center of each cell. This protein then moves to the cell wall and acts like a tunnel for chloride to pass through.

Where Do My Genes Come From?

You may be wondering why you have your father's nose but your brother has your mother's nose. Well, when a baby is born it gets twenty-three chromosomes—or strings of genes—from each parent. Each parent gives his or her child only half of his or her genes. A baby is born with a full set of genes, half from the mother and half from the father. This way, no two people are exactly alike, not even brothers and sisters. Only identical twins have exactly the same genes as each other.

To have cystic fibrosis, people have to have two defective CFTR genes. They have to get one copy of the gene from their father and one from their mother. People who have only one copy of the defective gene don't have cystic fibrosis. That is because the CFTR gene is recessive. When genes pair up, sometimes one gene is dominant, or stronger, than the other gene. The normal CFTR gene is dominant. This means that when it pairs up with a defective gene, the normal gene is what the body listens to. For the recessive gene to control the body, the normal, dominant gene must be absent.

People who have one normal gene and one defective one are called carriers. If two carriers have a child, there is a one-in-four, or 25 percent, chance that their child will have CF. There is a 50 percent chance that their child will be a carrier, and there is a 25 percent chance that their child won't get a copy of the defective gene and won't be a carrier.

Every child gets a completely new set of genes. So it doesn't matter if one child in a family has CF. If both parents are carriers, the second child will still have a 25 percent chance of getting it. About one out of every thirty white Americans is a carrier of CF. This means that about one out of every 3,600 babies is born with cystic fibrosis.

Chapter Three | How Is Cystic Fibrosis Diagnosed and Treated?

Because people who are carriers don't have cystic fibrosis, they usually don't even know that they are carriers. If they don't know that they are carriers, then they don't suspect that their child has CF. So how do people know if they or their children have CF?

The Symptoms

Many times, the problems that CF causes are not obvious until later in life. Children with a mild case of CF may cough a lot and have trouble with chest infections, but many children have these problems. Sometimes doctors don't know that they should be looking for CF because it isn't in the family medical history. Of course, sometimes the symptoms are obvious. One of the symptoms of babies with CF is jaundiced, or yellowish, skin. Another occasional symptom of newborns with CF is a clogged intestine. Doctors can usually clear this problem without surgery, but sometimes they actually have to surgically unblock the intestine.

However, these symptoms don't occur in every child with CF. Another clue is that as children with CF get older, they tend to have many problems with respiratory infections, pneumonia, and chronic bronchitis. Eighty-five percent of people with CF also have digestive troubles and may eat a ton of food but never seem to gain weight.

One common symptom of people with cystic fibrosis is extremely salty sweat. This was discovered one hot summer in New York City. Now this symptom is one of the major ways of telling whether someone has the disease or not.

The Sweat Test

The summer sun beat down. It baked the black asphalt of the streets of New York City. Heat waves shimmered in the distance. The light glinted off of windshields and rooftops. Kids played ball in the basketball courts and guzzled water and sweated like crazy. Some children even fainted. It was the summer of 1952. Many of the children who fainted ended up in the hospital. Many of them had cystic fibrosis.

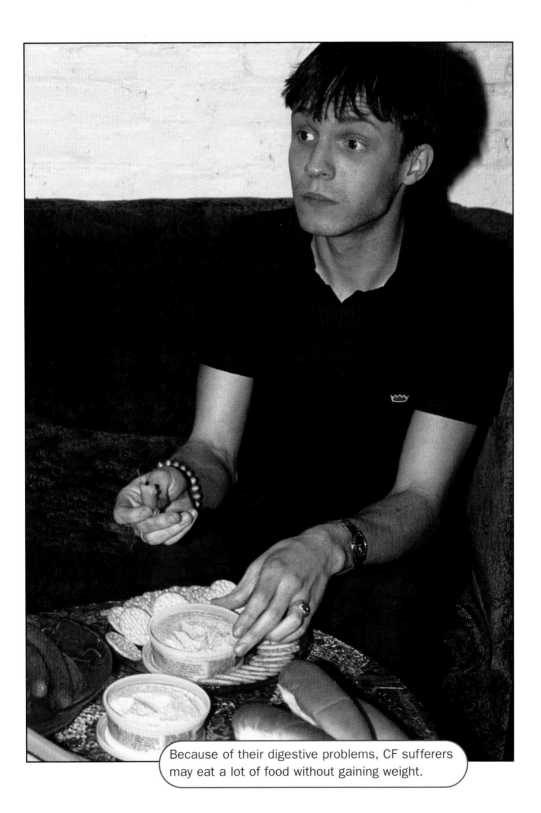
Because of their digestive problems, CF sufferers may eat a lot of food without gaining weight.

People with CF have a harder time staying hydrated (keeping water in their bodies) than do most people because their skin can't reabsorb the salt that is needed. When these children ended up in the hospital, doctors at the Columbia University College of Physicians and Surgeons noticed that the kids all had very salty sweat. This was an important discovery, and now doctors perform sweat tests to see if a person has CF.

To perform the sweat test, doctors put a drug called pilocarpine on the person's forearm. This drug makes the sweat glands produce sweat. The doctors pass a mild electric current across the skin to make it absorb the drug. Then they put a piece of filter paper on the skin and absorb the sweat. The paper is sent to the lab to determine how much salt is in the sweat. People with CF have two to five times the amount of salt in their sweat as people without the disease.

Genetic Testing

Now that scientists have discovered the gene that carries CF, they can test for the disease genetically. To do this, they scrape cells from the cheek of a patient and examine the DNA of the cells to see if a defective CFTR gene is there.

This test isn't always accurate because it doesn't test for all the different problems that cause CF. There are over 700 ways that the gene can be defective and any one of these defects can cause CF. The genetic test can detect only about seventy of these major defects. Scientists are working on a test that will detect eighty-six of the major defects. As of now, genetic testing identifies only three out of every four individuals with CF. To be sure about the diagnosis, doctors often use genetic testing along with the sweat test.

Treating Cystic Fibrosis

Once a person is diagnosed with CF, treatment can begin right away.

The Use of Exercise

Exercise is important to us because it is one of the ways in which we take care of our bodies. Exercise is even more important to people with cystic fibrosis. Aerobic exercise, the kind that makes your heart beat faster, moves a lot of air through your lungs. This is really good for people with CF. It makes the body more efficient at getting oxygen out of the air and into the blood. It also expands the lungs, making them capable of holding more air. Lots of aerobic exercise helps to keep the lungs free of infections. The flow of air through the lungs also helps to break up the sticky mucus and get it out of the body.

Nonaerobic exercise, such as weight lifting, is useful, too, because the heart doesn't have to work as hard to move the blood around. Exercise also has a psychological benefit; it makes people feel good about themselves.

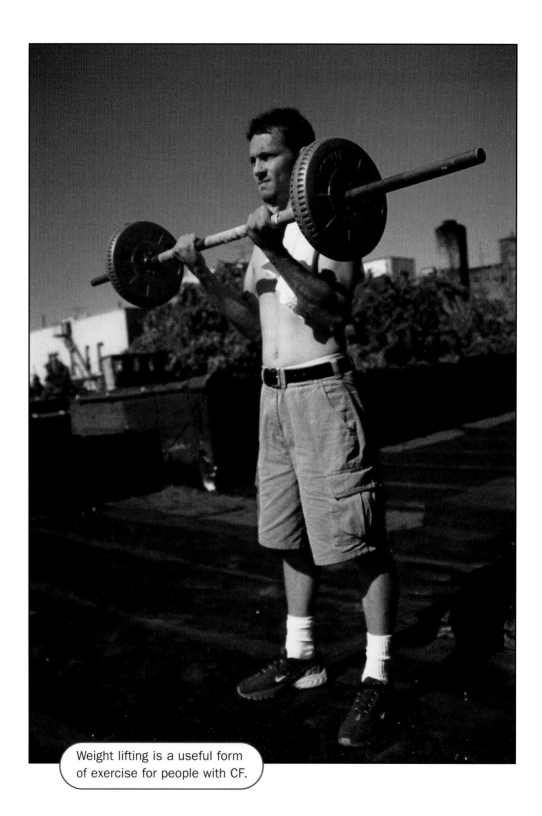

Weight lifting is a useful form of exercise for people with CF.

There is no type of exercise that is better than another for people with cystic fibrosis. Doctors recommend doing activities that are enjoyable. People with CF participate in all sorts of competitive and noncompetitive sports. However, they do need to be careful of dehydration, especially in extremely hot, humid weather. Just like everybody else, people with CF should stop exercising if they feel lightheaded or have difficulty breathing.

Diet and Nutrition

Food is as important to life as air and water. Unfortunately, we don't always eat the right foods. Just like everyone else, people with CF need to get enough nutrients from their food in order to maintain a healthy body. Also, those with CF need to get enough food so that their lungs have the energy needed to fight infections. Because of digestive problems, those with CF may have trouble getting nutrients from the food they eat.

Usually people with this disease eat a normal, healthy diet that is supplemented with enzymes—special chemicals that help digest the food. These enzymes come in capsules or little granules. The capsules are coated with a special substance that keeps them safe in the stomach. Once they reach the intestine, they open up and help digest the food. The enzymes should be taken before or during meals and snacks. It is important not to take them with milk because milk eats through the protective coating of the capsule.

Sometimes people with CF can't get enough nutrients even with the extra enzymes. In this case, eating high-energy foods like milkshakes might help. If not, a small tube may have to be inserted into the stomach. This tube is used to put high-calorie food directly into the stomach, usually at night while the person sleeps.

Physical Therapy for the Lungs—Physiotherapy

Physiotherapy can be used specifically to help keep the lungs healthy and clear of mucus. Thick mucus gets clogged in the lungs, causing all sorts of problems. Physiotherapy attacks these problems by helping to get the mucus out of the lungs.

Physiotherapy consists of banging or thumping certain areas of the chest, loosening the mucus so that it can drain out of the lungs. The patient lies in a certain position so that gravity can help drain the lungs. The person receiving the treatment can help by coughing and breathing deeply and quickly.

Usually physiotherapy is done twice a day—in the morning and the evening—for half an hour each time. Morning therapy is especially important because it helps the body rid itself of the mucus that has built up during the night. Physiotherapy should not be done right after eating because it can make a person vomit. Right after therapy is the time to take any inhaled antibiotics or medicines because they can better reach the areas of the lungs that they have to get to.

If a person is sick and has extra mucus in his or her lungs, physiotherapy may be done more than twice a day or for longer periods of time. Doctors have many tests that they can do to see how the different areas of the lungs are doing. If one is more clogged than another, that area may need special attention. One of the tests doctors use to determine how the lungs are doing is called a chest scan. During a chest scan, the patient inhales a harmless, radioactive gas. The gas shows up on special tools that are sensitive to radiation, and the doctor can tell what areas of the lungs need attention. Doctors also use X rays and more traditional tests to monitor the respiratory system.

For those who don't want to depend on others for help, there are tools that allow them to perform self-physiotherapy. One of these tools is a vibrating vest or pack. Doctors who specialize in cystic fibrosis will be able to tell you all about other interesting tools that help with physiotherapy. Your doctor should also be able to tell you where to get these tools.

A new part of physiotherapy is the use of D-Nase, a drug that was approved in 1994. D-Nase helps break up the mucus in the lungs of certain people with CF. The drug is expensive and is taken through a nebulizer, a special machine used for taking inhaled drugs. People with CF may want to ask their doctors whether or not D-Nase is a good idea for them.

Fighting Infections

Cystic fibrosis alone is a problem, but it gets really harmful when it is combined with infections in the lungs. The thick mucus associated with CF makes it hard for white blood cells to do their job and keeps bacteria-infected mucus in the lungs. It also puts a general strain on the immune system by making it harder for the body to get nutrients and vitamins and to fight infections. When infections occur, especially in the lungs, they can cause permanent damage and scarring. This can lead to a decreased ability to breathe.

Antibiotics

Overall health is a good tool in the fight against infections. So is a positive attitude. Another important tool doctors use to fight infections is antibiotics. Antibiotics are drugs that help the body kill unwanted bacteria. They are like extra soldiers for your body's army. Your body produces antibiotics, but sometimes they aren't enough, or in the case of people with cystic fibrosis, they are ineffective.

To help people with cystic fibrosis fight infections, doctors prescribe a variety of antibiotics. They come in the form of pills, tablets, liquids, and mists that are inhaled. The problem with antibiotics is that sometimes bacteria can become resistant to them. When this occurs, the antibiotics can't kill the bacteria anymore. It is important to finish the whole prescription when you

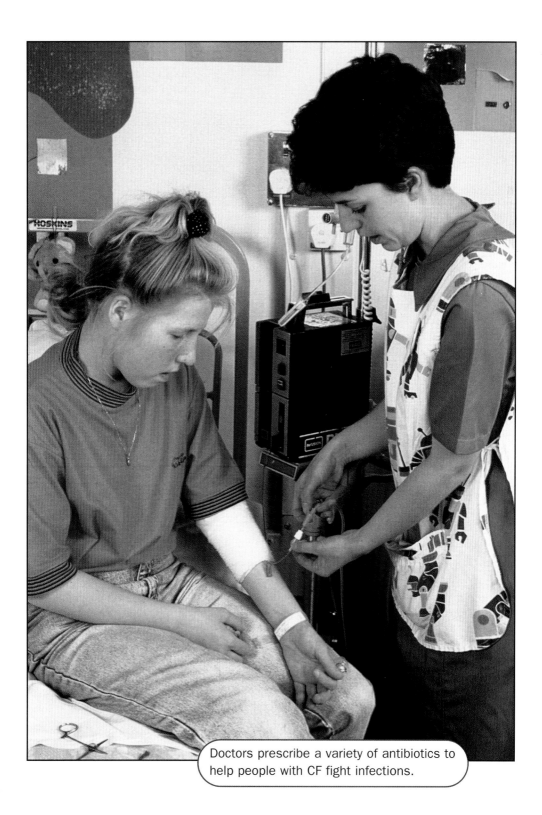

Doctors prescribe a variety of antibiotics to help people with CF fight infections.

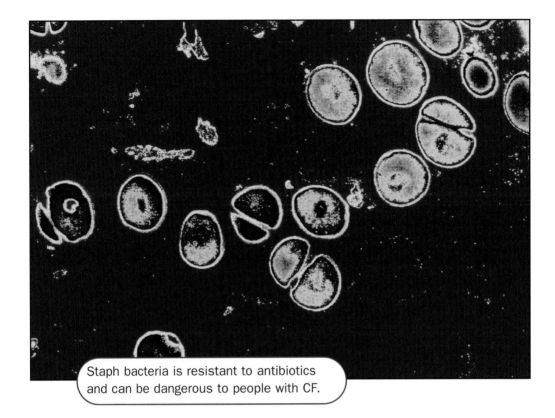

Staph bacteria is resistant to antibiotics and can be dangerous to people with CF.

take antibiotics. Otherwise, there may be some bacteria left that can develop new armor and not be hurt by the drugs anymore, and you can become reinfected.

One kind of bacteria that is resistant to antibiotics is called *P. cepacia*. Doctors don't have any antibiotics that can kill this bacteria. Once it gets into the lungs of a person with CF, it never leaves and can cause serious damage to the lungs. Because there is no way to kill it, many CF clinics treat people with *P. cepacia* separately from other patients so that the bacteria won't spread. *P. cepacia* is not a problem for people without CF, so contact with doctors, family, and friends usually isn't an issue.

One other bacteria that has been known to beat antibiotics is called staph. This is a bacteria that lives on our skin and is usually not harmful. In people with CF, however, it can cause lung infections. These infections are usually treated with an antibiotic called methicillin. Unfortunately, there are now some types of this bacteria that have figured out how to beat the antibiotic. They are called methicillin resistant staphylococcus aureus, or MRSA. CF patients with MRSA are encouraged to avoid contact with other people with CF because the resistant bacteria can be passed from person to person. Like *P. cepacia,* MRSA is not a health problem for people without cystic fibrosis. To fight infections in people who have CF, doctors often prescribe two different antibiotics at the same time. This helps because the double dosage kills the bacteria before they can figure out how to beat both antibiotics.

Lung Transplants

Eventually the lungs of people with CF may get so bad that they can no longer breathe. When this happens, they can actually get a new pair of lungs. Scientists have been performing lung transplants in the United States since 1985. But even though lung transplants are an option, they are not always the easiest solution.

The Last Alternative

When there is no other way to keep a CF patient healthy, lung transplants are performed as a last alternative. The good news is that once the donated lungs

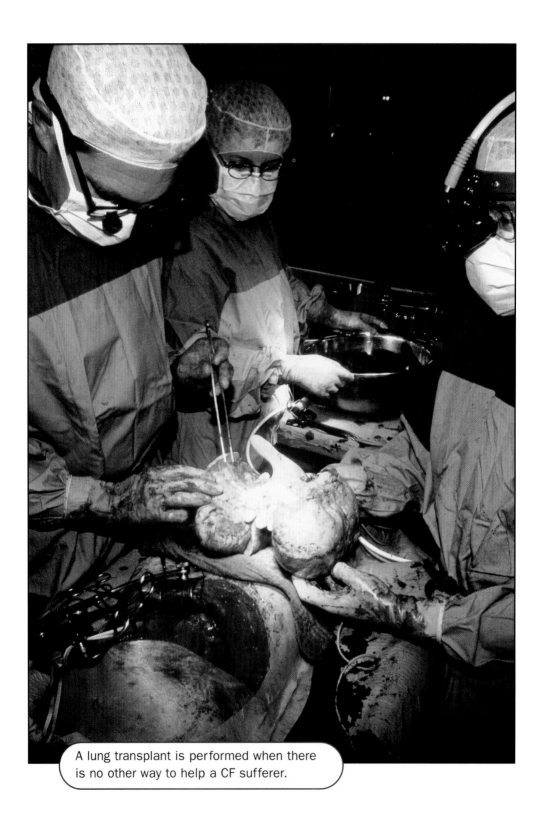

A lung transplant is performed when there is no other way to help a CF sufferer.

are inside a CF sufferer, they will continue to make CFTR. This means that the new lungs won't have CF and the mucus produced inside them will be normal. Of course, patients will still have CF, their sweat will still be salty, and they will still have to take enzymes to digest their food, but their new lungs will be healthy.

The problem with lung transplants is that the body doesn't always accept them. People who have transplants have to take drugs called immunosuppressants. These drugs stop the immune system from attacking the new lungs. Unfortunately, they also stop the immune system from attacking the bacteria and viruses it needs to fight. This is why, after a transplant, a patient has to be extra careful of infections.

Another problem with this surgery is finding a suitable pair of lungs. People who are alive need their lungs, and once someone dies the lungs can be kept alive only for a short period of time. There is a long waiting list for lung transplants, and people with CF aren't the only people waiting for lungs. Many people who have hurt their lungs by smoking also need new lungs. Also, not everyone who dies donates his or her lungs. A lot of people don't realize how important it is to be a donor.

Improvements in Transplants

More than 70 percent of patients survive the first year after a lung transplant. It is also encouraging that the waiting list for donor lungs is getting shorter, meaning that people are waiting less time to have this potentially life-saving operation. It is about eighteen months from the time a person gets on a waiting list to the time he or she gets a transplant.

As with most things, doctors find that the people who do the best after surgery are the ones who stay healthy, have a positive attitude, and have family and friends to help them. Some people find that after the surgery they can bike, run, skate, return to work, and live completely normal lives.

There is one other fairly new procedure that is being tried. Some people are getting lung transplants from living donors. To do this, there have to be two donors. Every person has five lobes, or sections, of lung, two on one side of the chest and three on the other. Each donor gives two lobes to the patient, leaving himself or herself with three healthy lobes. The patient receives four new lobes. This is complicated because it involves three people who have to undergo surgery. It is also trickier because the donor lungs have to match each other. Usually they come from close relatives.

Chapter Four

How Does Cystic Fibrosis Affect Your Life?

One of the most common questions people ask is how cystic fibrosis will affect their lives. Two groups of people ask this question: those who have the disease, and those who know people who have CF. Some CF sufferers have it from birth. They learn from the time they are babies how the disease affects their lives. For parents and friends of these people, the disease can come as more of a shock. Sometimes CF isn't diagnosed until people are older, and in that case, they must start from the beginning and figure out how the disease affects their lives and how they can best cope with it.

The Sky Is the Limit

People who have cystic fibrosis do die; ultimately, the disease is fatal. However, people with CF are living longer and healthier lives than CF sufferers used to. People who live with cystic fibrosis need to take special care of themselves, but they don't need to feel that they can't do things that other people do. There is no activity or lifestyle that is out of the question for someone with CF. However, there are some very real ways the disease impacts their existence. An awareness of these issues can help people deal with them in a more effective way.

Some Real Considerations

People with CF do all sorts of sports and activities, and they have all sorts of jobs. People should not let the disease dictate their lives. Friends and family of people with CF shouldn't treat them any differently than any other person they care about and love.

Medicine and Physiotherapy

People with cystic fibrosis often need to take a lot of medicine, and they need to have physiotherapy every day. These are not major problems, they just require a little bit of planning. Many people find that making physiotherapy fun, by doing it while watching television or listening to music, for example, helps make it an accepted part of their daily routines. Medicine is another thing that needs to be a part of the day-to-day routine. Many people with CF carry extra pills with them. This way, in case they forget to take pills, they will not run into problems.

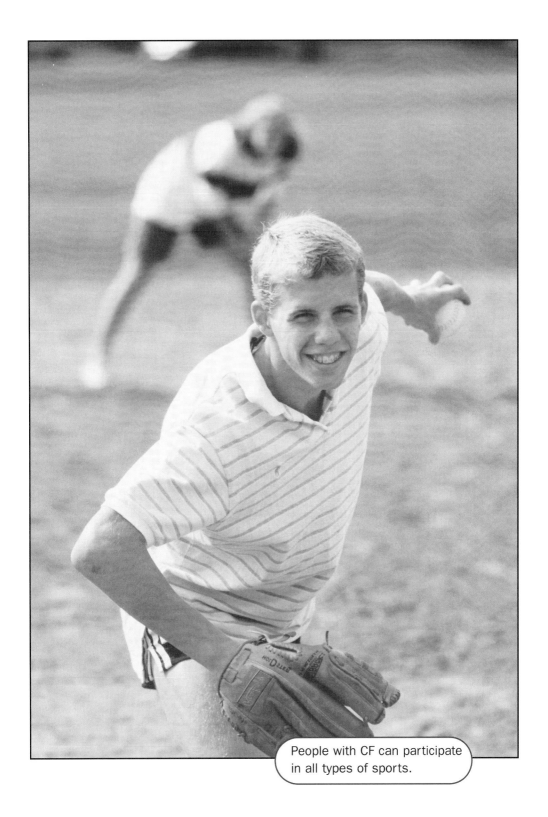

People with CF can participate in all types of sports.

Sometimes pills can be mixed into food to make them easier to take. People with CF must be sure to plan ahead before traveling or changing their normal routines. Traveling smartly involves packing enough medicine and figuring out how to do physiotherapy in a different place, sometimes without the help of friends or family.

Embarrassing Odors

We have already mentioned that people with CF have salty sweat. This is not a problem, but often they also have extremely bad-smelling stool. This is a potentially embarrassing issue. Many people find that carrying a book of matches helps. After using the rest room they light a few matches. The burning sulfur neutralizes the smell. This is handy on airplanes or while staying at a friend's house.

Dealing with Hospitalization

Cystic fibrosis is a serious disease, and people who suffer from it may have to spend time in the hospital. Being aware of this fact makes it easier to deal with. Employers, teachers, and even friends should know about this possibility, so that when it happens people can deal with the absence. Schoolwork can be brought to the person in the hospital so he or she doesn't fall behind. Another thing that helps with hospital visits is to have a bag packed or a checklist of things to bring. Favorite toys, books, or movies can make time in a hospital go more quickly. Many hospitals offer fun

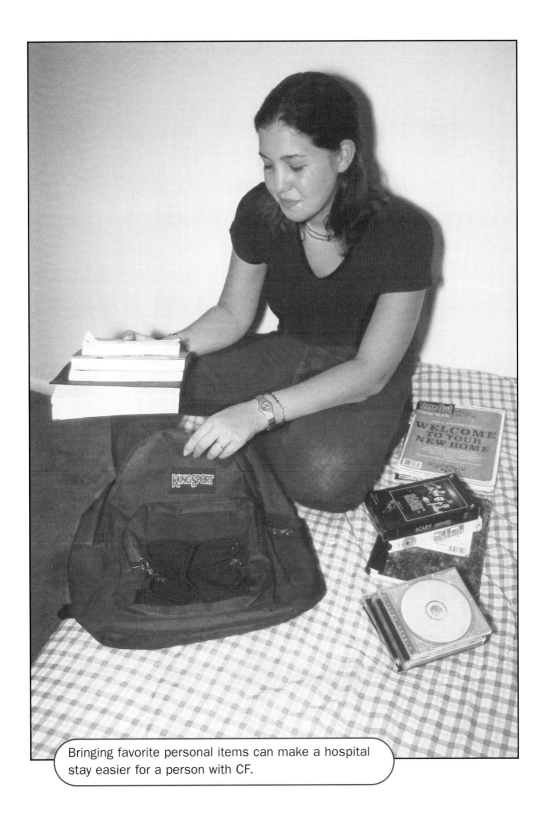

Bringing favorite personal items can make a hospital stay easier for a person with CF.

things to do while you are there. Be sure to ask the staff what activities there are to do.

Children—To Have or Not to Have?

One of the major concerns facing people with cystic fibrosis is the decision whether or not to have children and risk having a child with CF. If a person with CF has a child, the child will at least be a carrier of the disease. If the spouse isn't a carrier, then the child will definitely not have CF. But if the spouse is a carrier, then the child will have a 75 percent chance of being born with the disease.

Many times, it may be harder for these couples to have children because males with CF tend to be infertile. However, thanks to modern science this isn't necessarily a problem. If a male with CF wants to have a child, doctors can take sperm from him and fertilize an egg with it. Likewise, females who have trouble becoming pregnant because of their disease can seek help through artificial insemination, a process that helps the sperm reach the egg.

Adoption is another way to have a child, but many people with CF worry that they may not be healthy enough to provide all the care a child needs while growing up. Some people feel that they don't want to have a child if their health is questionable. Remember, for people with CF, death is a very real possibility. These are

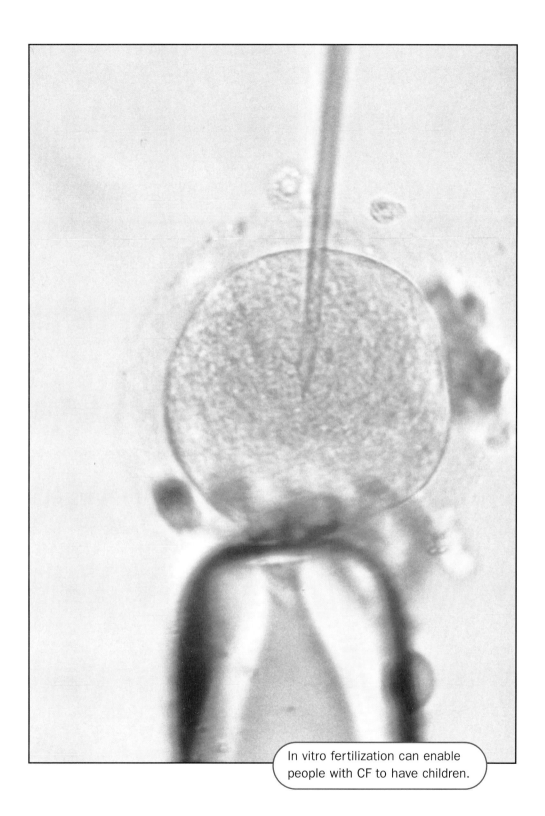

In vitro fertilization can enable people with CF to have children.

all issues that people with CF have to consider before deciding to have and raise children.

Coping with a Fatal Disease

Dealing with a fatal disease is not easy. Different people deal with it in varying ways. Some people turn to religion or find comfort in spirituality. Other people want to learn everything they can about the science of the illness. Some people use humor to deal with it; they find that if they can joke about the problem, it doesn't seem quite as scary. Some people see it as a challenge that needs to be conquered. Most people try not to let the disease run their lives.

Anyway you choose to look at it, cystic fibrosis is a hard thing to deal with, both for the people who have it and for those who care about them. The one thing that seems to be true is that a positive attitude helps the situation.

Siblings of Cystic Fibrosis Sufferers

Sometimes brothers and sisters of people with cystic fibrosis have a particularly hard time coping with the disease. Younger siblings may not understand why their parents have to spend so much time with the sick person. One way for parents to solve this problem is by including the nonsick sibling in more of what is going on, asking how he or she feels, explaining problems, and having him or her help with administering medicine or the physiotherapy.

Sometimes siblings experience feelings of guilt because they are healthy and their brother or sister is sick. This is normal. The best way to deal with it is to discuss it so everyone understands that it isn't anyone's fault. Siblings naturally worry about losing their brother or sister. This is a very real fear. There is no easy way around this, but discussion can help people deal with these feelings of fear.

Too Much Attention

Parents and loved ones worry about people who have health problems. Those with cystic fibrosis need to understand that this worry is natural. The person with CF may get tired of explaining to friends or others how the disease works, or how he or she is feeling. He or she may also become tired of the sympathy and extra attention that ill people receive. Not everyone likes getting a lot of attention; it can be stifling. Also, friends and family members should be sensitive to the fact that people with diseases don't want to spend all of their time talking about their illness.

Talking It Out—Beyond Your Family

When people do need to talk about their emotions, and they don't want to speak with their families, there are places to go and get help. Many people go to professional counselors to help them look at the problem in a different way. There are support groups for people with cystic fibrosis and their families. There

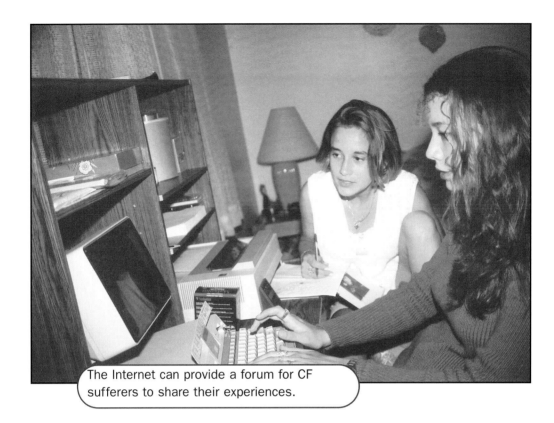

The Internet can provide a forum for CF sufferers to share their experiences.

are also Internet forums and sites that let people share their experiences and relate to others' stories. The Where to Go for Help section at the back of this book lists a lot of information on associations that are there to help CF patients and their families.

Chapter Five | A Glimpse into the Future

The future outlook is good for people with cystic fibrosis. Scientists are learning more and more about this disease. They are experimenting with new drugs and therapies, and looking for new cures. There are many groups that provide scientists with money so that they can continue their work. This chapter deals with some of the newer possibilities for treating cystic fibrosis.

Gene Therapy

Science has only recently discovered how genes work. In 1989, scientists isolated the gene responsible for CF. This development has opened the door to a world of treatment possibilities that we are only beginning to explore. Many people hope one day to solve the problem of CF by replacing the genes of people with the disease with normal genes. This is called gene therapy.

Each cell carries genes—or strings of information—inside it. This information tells the cell how to work. If we could somehow figure out how to change the information inside the cells of people with CF, then those cells would work normally. That is why when a person gets a lung transplant, the new lungs don't get the disease because those cells know how to work correctly.

Gene therapy is a new science. Scientists have been able to change the genes of cells in the laboratory. The problem is how to change the genes of the lung cells in people with CF. To get the new genes into the cells, many scientists hope to use viruses. Viruses are tiny organisms that get inside cells. Once a virus gets inside a cell, it takes over and replaces the cell's gene information with its own. Some viruses are harmful and can make us sick. Scientists are experimenting with using a virus that causes the common cold to deliver the gene therapy.

Why Gene Therapy Is Problematic

There are some problems with gene therapy. Often the body of the person attacks the virus delivering the gene therapy because it thinks it is dangerous. It also attacks the cells that the virus infects, the very cells that need to be saved. Another problem is that cells regularly die and are replaced. In CF sufferers, the cells are replaced by

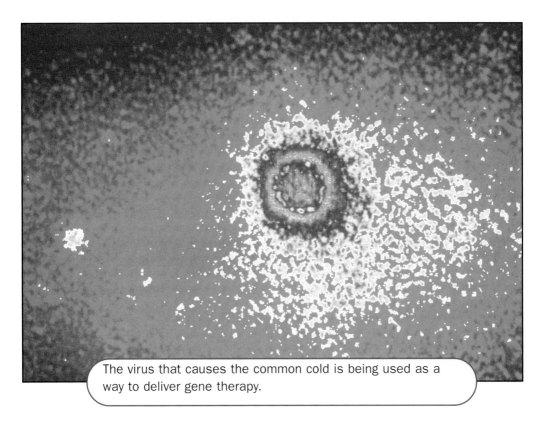

The virus that causes the common cold is being used as a way to deliver gene therapy.

ones that have the wrong information. This means that gene therapy would probably have to be repeated every few months so that there would be enough cells with the right information to keep the person healthy. Scientists are experimenting with gene therapy now and hopefully this new science will help people with cystic fibrosis.

Other Possible Therapies

There are other therapies for cystic fibrosis that are being developed. One of these is the use of new drugs to help the cells of the person make a tunnel for chloride to pass through. This would solve the problem of CF and allow the salt in the cells to pass freely.

47

Another thing scientists are trying to do is work with the tools the body already has. One of the major problems with CF sufferers is that their immune systems can't kill the infections that occur in the lungs. This is because the sticky, salty mucus kills the natural antibiotic that should be fighting infections.

A couple of years ago, scientists figured out what this antibiotic is. Now they hope to change it so it can survive in the salty mucus of the lungs of a person with CF. If scientists can do this, then people with CF would have a very valuable tool in their battle against lung infections.

Xenotransplantation

We mentioned before how much lung transplants can help people with CF, but there aren't enough lungs to go around. One idea that is being worked on is the use of animal lungs in humans. This is called xenotransplantation. If scientists could use animal lungs, then there would be enough lungs to give transplants to everyone who needed them. Also, it could be timed so that the lungs would be fresh when they were transplanted. However, many people feel that xenotransplantation is unfair to animals.

Hope for the Future

Whatever you think of these different possible therapies, one thing for sure is that there is a lot of hope for people with CF. There are many scientists working on finding better treatments and even a cure for this disease. With every new advance, people with cystic fibrosis live longer, healthier, more complete lives. When you remember that only thirty years ago, most people with CF didn't live to adulthood, what has been accomplished is amazing.

In the last fifteen years, scientists have figured out how to do lung transplants, which gene CF is on, and how to change genetic information. New drugs and machines are available and more are coming. There is more reason than ever to keep a positive attitude.

Glossary

alveoli   Small sacs in the lungs that absorb oxygen into the blood and push out carbon dioxide.

antibiotic   Substance produced either by the body or synthetically that inhibits or kills microorganisms.

artificial insemination   Scientific method for helping people have babies. It involves the mechanical placement of sperm in a woman's uterus.

bacteria   Small, one-celled organisms that can cause disease.

bile   Greenish yellow liquid produced by the liver that helps the body break down fats.

CFTR   Cystic fibrosis transmembrane conductance regulator. This protein acts like a tunnel through cell walls, allowing chloride ions to pass through.

chromosome   Threadlike structure that carries genes from the parent to the child. Chromosomes are made of DNA.

cilia   Tiny, hairlike projections that line certain parts of the body.

cirrhosis   Condition caused when a person's liver is damaged and doesn't work properly.

DNA   Deoxyribonucleic acid. DNA is the material that genes and chromosomes are made out of.

enzyme   Protein that speeds up chemical processes in the body. Many enzymes are used by the body to digest food.

epithelial cells   Small cells that line parts of the body.

gene   One unit of heredity. One piece of information that is passed on from parent to child. Genes are made of DNA and are carried on chromosomes.

gene therapy   Inserting normal genes into cells to replace damaged genes in order to treat a disease.

immunosuppressants   Drugs that keep the body from attacking bacteria, viruses, and other foreign bodies.

intestine   Place in the body where the final digestion and absorption of food occurs after it has passed through the stomach.

ion   Atom that has either lost or gained electrons, giving it an electric charge.

mucous cells   Small cells that line parts of the body and produce mucus.

mucus   Slippery secretion of the body that helps to moisten and protect certain body parts.

pancreas   Gland in human beings that produces many enzymes that aid in the digestion of food.

protein   Small compound that the body uses to make cells and other structures. We get proteins from the food we eat.

starch   Type of food that the body needs. Starches are broken down into sugars by the digestive system.

stool   The solid waste product produced by the body; excrement.

transplant   Operation in which an organ or part of the body is taken from one person and put into another.

viruses   Simple microorganisms that can cause infection.

xenotransplantation   The use of animal parts in human transplant operations.

Where to Go for Help

In the United States

Boomer Esiason Foundation
One World Trade Center
101st Floor
New York, NY 10048
(212) 938-4376 or (800) 789-4376
http://www.esiason.org/
Football star Boomer Esiason's son, Gunnar, has CF.
This Web site and foundation do a lot to fund research
and provide information about the disease.

Cystic Fibrosis Foundation
6931 Arlington Road
Bethesda, MD 20814
(301) 951-4422

(800) FIGHT CF (344-4823)
http://www.cff.org/
You can find just about any information you want
about CF at this site. It is also a great place to turn for
help when you need it.

Cystic Fibrosis Research, Inc.
560 San Antonio Road, Suite 103
Palo Alto, CA 94306-4349
(650) 856-0546
http://www.cfri.org/
This site is very technical but is a great place to learn
more about the disease. It also has a wonderful new
searchable database of information.

National Center for Biotechnology Information
National Library of Medicine
Building 38A, Room 8N805
Bethesda, MD 20894
(301) 496-2475
http://www.ncbi.nlm.nih.gov/cgi-bin/SCIENCE96/
nph-gene?CFTR
The National Center for Biotechnology Information
Web site offers an overview of how the gene in cystic
fibrosis works.

National Institutes of Health
National Heart, Lung, and Blood Institute
P.O. Box 30105
Bethesda, MD 20824-0105
(301) 592-8573
http://www.nhlb.nih.gov/health/public/lung/other/cf.htm
Facts about cystic fibrosis.

In Canada

Canadian Cystic Fibrosis Foundation
2221 Yonge Street, Suite 601
Toronto, ON M4S 2B4
(416) 485-9149 or (800) 378-CCFF (2233)
http://www.ccff.ca

The Canadian Lung Association
3 Raymond Street, Suite 300
Ottawa, ON K1R 1A3
(613) 569-6411
http://www.lung.ca
A site dedicated to healthy lungs.

Manitoba Lung Association
629 McDermot Avenue, 2nd Floor
Winnipeg, MB R3A 1P6
(204) 774-5501
http://www.mb.lung.ca/

Niagara Cystic Fibrosis Chapter
http://www.iaw.on.ca/~meb/

Web Sites

CF Online Index
http://vmsb.csd.mu.edu/~5418lukasr/cystic.html
This site is a great place to explore cystic fibrosis on the
Web. It has just about every on-line resource available.

CF-Web
http://cf-web.mit.edu/
This is a great place to start. It offers some basic defi-
nitions of the disease as well as many links to other
cool sites.

CysticFibrosis.com
http://www.cysticfibrosis.com/
An Internet community for cystic fibrosis patients,
families, and loved ones.

Cystic-L CF Information and Support
http://www.cystic-l.org/
This is a wonderful place to meet people who have and
know people with CF. There are recent articles on the
disease, discussion forums, pictures of people with the
disease, and a shop to buy CF-related items.

The Kids Health Homepage
http://www.kidshealth.org/
Kids Health is a great place to find simple information about many health concerns.

The University of Wisconsin's CF page
http://www2.medsch.wisc.edu/childrenshosp/CF/cf.html
This site is a little more technical. It offers up-to-date information about the disease and about its clinic and what it is doing.

For Further Reading

Bryan, Jenny. *Breathing: The Respiratory System.* New York: Dillon Press, 1993.

Chumbley, Jane. *Cystic Fibrosis: A Family Affair.* London: SPCK and Triangle, 1999.

Cook, Allen R., and Peter D. Dresser, eds. *Respiratory Diseases and Disorders Sourcebook.* Detroit, MI: Omnigraphics, 1995.

Deford, Frank. *Alex: The Life of a Child.* Nashville, TN: Rutledge Hill Press, 1997.

Grishaw, Joshua. *My Heart Is Full of Wishes.* Chatham, NJ: Raintree Steck-Vaughn, 2000.

Harris, Ann, and Maurice Super. *Cystic Fibrosis: The Facts.* New York: Oxford University Press, 1995.

Hopkin, Karen. *Understanding Cystic Fibrosis.* Jackson, MS: University Press of Mississippi, 1998.

Lindy, Burton. *The Family Life of Sick Children.* London: Routledge & Kegan Paul, 1975.

Orenstein, David M. *Cystic Fibrosis: A Guide for Patient and Family.* Philadelphia: Lippincott-Raven Publishers, 1997.

Parker, Steve. *The Lungs and Respiratory System.* Chatham, NJ: Raintree Steck-Vaughn, 1997.

Silverstein, Alvin, Robert Silverstein, and Virginia B. Silverstein. *Cystic Fibrosis.* Danbury, CT: Franklin Watts, 1994.

Wine, Jeffrey. *CFTR and the Molecular Basis of Cystic Fibrosis.* London: Chapman and Hall, 1998.

Index

About the Author

Justin Lee lives and works in New York City. He has been acquainted with a person living with cystic fibrosis for many years now. This person has made the world a better place.

Photo Credits

Cover and p. 29 © Custom Medical/Science Photo Library; p. 2 © Simon Fraser/Science Photo Library; p. 11 © Custom Medical/J. L. Carson; p. 13 © Alex Grey/Peter Arnold, Inc.; pp. 16, 47 © Custom Medical Stock Photo; p. 21 by Simca Israelian; p. 24 by Louis Dollagory; p. 30 © Custom Medical/J. L. Carson; p. 32 © Argus Fotoarchive/Peter Arnold, Inc.; p. 37 © SuperStock, Inc.; p. 39 by Shalhevet Moshe; p. 41 © Custom Medical/Richard B. Rawlins; p. 44 by Maria Moreno.